CHAIR YOGA
MASTERY

ELEVATE AT 60+

HENRY I. GREAT

Copyright © 2024 by Henry I. Great

All rights reserved. No part of this publication may be reproduced, distributed, or transmitted in any form or by any means, including photocopying, recording, or other electronic or mechanical methods, without the prior written permission of the publisher, except in the case of brief quotations embodied in critical reviews and certain other noncommercial uses permitted by copyright law.

TABLE OF CONTENTS

CHAPTER ONE 6

1.1 INTRODUCTION 6

1.2 Setting the Stage: Explaining the benefits and accessibility of chair yoga for seniors. 7

1.3 Personal Journey: Share a brief personal anecdote or journey with chair yoga. 9

1.4 Understanding Chair Yoga: Defining chair yoga and its relevance for seniors. 11

CHAPTER TWO 13

2.1 THE FOUNDATIONS OF CHAIR YOGA 13

2.2 Exploring the Basics: Detailed Explanation of Chair Yoga Poses, Modifications, and Props 15

2.3 Safety First: Tips for Practicing Safely and Effectively in Chair Yoga 18

2.4 Setting Up Your Space: Guidance on Creating a Comfortable and Conducive Environment for Practice 21

CHAPTER THREE 24

3.1 CHAIR YOGA FOR MOBILITY AND FLEXIBILITY 24

3.2 Gentle Warm-Ups: Sequences Focusing on Loosening Stiff Joints and Improving Flexibility 27

3.3 Mobility Boosters: Exercises to Enhance Range of Motion and Ease Everyday Movements 30

3.4 Targeted Stretches: Techniques for Specific Areas like Hips, Shoulders, and Spine 33

CHAPTER FOUR **36**

4.1 CHAIR YOGA FOR STRENGTH AND BALANCE **36**

4.2 Building Strength: Chair-Based Exercises to Improve Muscle Tone and Stability 39

4.3 Finding Balance: Practices to Enhance Equilibrium and Reduce the Risk of Falls 42

4.4 Core Connection: Strengthening the Core Muscles for Better Posture and Stability 46

CHAPTER FIVE **50**

5.1 CHAIR YOGA FOR MIND-BODY CONNECTION **50**

5.2 The Power of Breath: Deep Breathing Exercises for Relaxation and Stress Relief 53

5.3 Meditation in Motion: Incorporating Mindfulness into Chair Yoga Poses 57

5.4 Restorative Relaxation: Techniques for Deep Relaxation and Rejuvenation 60

CHAPTER SIX **64**

6.1 CHAIR YOGA FOR EVERYDAY WELLNESS **64**

6.2 Managing Chronic Conditions: Chair Yoga as a Complementary Therapy for Common Ailments like Arthritis and Osteoporosis 67

6.3 Improving Sleep: Relaxation Practices to Promote Better Sleep Quality 71

6.4 Enhancing Mental Clarity: Techniques for Sharpening Focus and Cognitive Function 74

CHAPTER SEVEN 77

   7.1 CHAIR YOGA FOR LIFE ENRICHMENT 77

      7.2 Chair Yoga in Community: Exploring Group Classes and the Social Benefits of Practicing Together 80

      7.3 Beyond the Chair: Adapting Chair Yoga Principles for Use in Daily Life 83

      7.4 Lifelong Practice: Encouragement for Maintaining a Consistent Chair Yoga Practice for Lifelong Well-Being 86

CHAPTER EIGHT 89

   8.1 CELEBRATING YOUR JOURNEY: REFLECTING ON THE TRANSFORMATIVE POWER OF CHAIR YOGA FOR SENIORS 89

      8.2 Continuing the Path: Resources for Further Exploration 92

      8.3 Gratitude and Farewell: Closing Thoughts and Well Wishes for Your Ongoing Wellness Journey 95

      Conclusion 97

CHAPTER ONE

1.1 INTRODUCTION

Welcome to the transformative world of chair yoga, where age is but a number and the possibilities for enhancing your well-being are endless. In this book, "Chair Yoga Mastery: Elevate Your Well-Being at 60+," we embark on a journey tailored specifically for seniors seeking to embrace the power of yoga from the comfort of their chairs.

As an experienced author and practitioner in the field of chair yoga, I understand the unique needs and desires of individuals aged 60 and above. This book is not just a guide; it's a testament to the remarkable potential within each of us to cultivate strength, flexibility, balance, and inner peace regardless of age or physical limitations.

Chair yoga offers a gentle yet powerful approach to fitness and mindfulness, making it accessible to everyone, regardless of fitness level or prior yoga experience. Whether you're recovering from an injury, managing a chronic condition, or simply looking to enhance your overall well-being, chair yoga provides a safe and effective means of achieving your goals.

In the following pages, we'll delve into the foundations of chair yoga, exploring essential techniques and principles to ensure a safe and fulfilling practice. From gentle stretches to dynamic movements, from soothing breathwork to profound relaxation, each chapter is designed to empower you on your journey to vitality and wholeness.

But this book is more than just a collection of poses and sequences; it's a celebration of community, connection, and the inherent joy of movement. Whether you're practicing alone in the comfort of your home or joining a group class in your local community center, know that you are part of a vibrant and supportive community of fellow seekers and practitioners.

So, I invite you to take a seat, open your heart, and embrace the possibilities that await you on this journey. Let "Chair Yoga Mastery" be your guide as you embark on a path of self-discovery, healing, and transformation. The chair is your sanctuary, the poses your allies, and the breath your constant companion. Together, let us elevate our well-being and embrace the fullness of life at 55 and beyond.

1.2 Setting the Stage: Explaining the benefits and accessibility of chair yoga for seniors.

As we embark on our journey into the world of chair yoga, it's essential to understand the profound benefits this practice offers and why it's uniquely suited for seniors. In this chapter, we'll explore the numerous advantages of chair yoga and highlight its accessibility for individuals of all ages and abilities.

1. **Gentle on the Joints**: One of the primary concerns for seniors is protecting their joints while staying active. Chair yoga provides a gentle, low-impact way to exercise, reducing the risk of strain or injury commonly associated with more vigorous forms of physical activity.
2. **Improved Flexibility and Mobility**: Aging often brings with it a natural decline in flexibility and mobility. Chair yoga offers a series of gentle stretches and movements designed to increase joint

mobility, enhance range of motion, and counteract the stiffness that can accompany aging.

3. **Enhanced Strength and Balance**: Maintaining muscle strength and balance is crucial for preventing falls and maintaining independence as we age. Chair yoga incorporates a variety of strength-building exercises that can be performed safely from a seated position, helping seniors build stability and confidence in their movements.

4. **Stress Reduction and Relaxation**: The practice of chair yoga emphasizes mindful breathing and relaxation techniques, which can help seniors manage stress, reduce anxiety, and promote a sense of calm and well-being. By learning to quiet the mind and release tension from the body, seniors can enjoy improved mental clarity and emotional resilience.

5. **Accessible to All Fitness Levels**: One of the most significant advantages of chair yoga is its accessibility. Whether you're a seasoned yogi or new to the practice, chair yoga can be adapted to meet your individual needs and abilities. With the use of props and modifications, participants can tailor each pose to suit their comfort level, ensuring a safe and enjoyable experience for all.

6. **Convenience and Comfort**: Unlike traditional yoga practices that require a large open space and specialized equipment, chair yoga can be practiced virtually anywhere, anytime. All you need is a sturdy chair and a small amount of floor space, making it an ideal option for seniors who may have mobility challenges or prefer the comfort and security of practicing at home.

By embracing the benefits of chair yoga, seniors can cultivate strength, flexibility, and inner peace, empowering themselves to live life to the fullest at any age. In the chapters that follow, we'll dive deeper into the techniques and practices that make chair yoga such a valuable tool for enhancing well-being and vitality in our senior years.

1.3 Personal Journey: Share a brief personal anecdote or journey with chair yoga.

My journey with chair yoga began at a time when I was searching for a gentle yet effective way to manage stress and improve my overall well-being. As a seasoned yoga practitioner, I had always appreciated the transformative power of yoga, but as life became busier and my body began to show signs of wear and tear, I found myself struggling to maintain a consistent practice.

It was during this time of reflection and self-discovery that I discovered chair yoga. At first, I'll admit, I was skeptical. How could sitting in a chair possibly provide the same benefits as traditional yoga on a mat? But as I began to explore this new approach to yoga, I quickly realized that chair yoga offered something truly unique and invaluable.

I'll never forget the first time I settled into my chair, closed my eyes, and took a deep breath. In that moment, I felt a profound sense of relaxation wash over me, as if the weight of the world had been lifted from my shoulders. As I moved through the gentle stretches and poses, I felt my body awaken and come alive in ways I hadn't experienced in years.

But it wasn't just the physical benefits of chair yoga that captivated me; it was the profound sense of peace and inner calm that I found with each practice. In the midst of life's chaos and uncertainty, chair yoga became my sanctuary, a place where I could find stillness amidst the storm and reconnect with the essence of who I truly am.

Through chair yoga, I discovered a newfound sense of strength, resilience, and self-compassion that continues to guide me on my journey to this day. It has taught me that yoga is not just about contorting your body into pretzel-like shapes; it's about embracing the fullness of life with an open heart and a mindful presence.

Now, as I share my passion for chair yoga with others, I am constantly inspired by the transformative power it holds for people of all ages and abilities. Whether you're recovering from an injury, managing a chronic condition, or simply seeking a gentle way to stay active and healthy, chair yoga offers a pathway to greater vitality, joy, and peace.

So, as you embark on your own journey with chair yoga, I invite you to open your heart, quiet your mind, and embrace the infinite possibilities that await you. May your practice be a source of strength, healing, and profound self-discovery, just as it has been for me.

1.4 Understanding Chair Yoga: Defining chair yoga and its relevance for seniors.

Chair yoga is a gentle yet powerful form of yoga that has been specifically adapted to accommodate individuals who may face challenges with mobility, balance, or flexibility, particularly seniors aged 55 and above. Unlike traditional yoga practices that typically involve standing or moving on a mat, chair yoga is performed primarily while seated or using a chair for support, making it accessible to a wide range of individuals.

At its core, chair yoga encompasses a variety of yoga poses, stretches, breathing exercises, and mindfulness practices that can be modified to suit the needs and abilities of seniors. By utilizing a chair as a stable prop, participants can safely engage in yoga postures and movements without the fear of losing balance or straining joints.

The relevance of chair yoga for seniors lies in its ability to address the unique physical, mental, and emotional needs that accompany aging:

1. **Physical Benefits**: Chair yoga offers numerous physical benefits for seniors, including improved flexibility, strength, balance, and joint mobility. Through gentle stretching and strengthening exercises, seniors can maintain or enhance their physical function, reducing the risk of falls and injuries while promoting overall health and vitality.

2. **Mind-Body Connection**: Chair yoga emphasizes the connection between breath, movement, and mindfulness, helping seniors cultivate greater body awareness and presence in the present moment. By focusing on the breath and practicing mindful

movement, seniors can reduce stress, anxiety, and depression, while enhancing mental clarity, focus, and emotional well-being.

3. **Adaptability and Accessibility**: One of the key advantages of chair yoga is its adaptability and accessibility for individuals of all fitness levels and abilities. Whether a senior is recovering from surgery, managing a chronic condition like arthritis or osteoporosis, or simply prefers a gentler approach to exercise, chair yoga offers a safe and effective way to stay active and healthy.

4. **Community and Social Connection**: Chair yoga provides seniors with an opportunity to connect with others in a supportive and inclusive environment. Group classes foster a sense of community, belonging, and camaraderie, reducing feelings of loneliness and isolation often experienced by older adults. Sharing the practice of chair yoga with peers can enhance motivation, accountability, and enjoyment, while fostering meaningful friendships and social connections.

In essence, chair yoga is more than just a form of exercise; it's a holistic approach to well-being that addresses the physical, mental, and emotional aspects of aging. By embracing chair yoga as part of their wellness routine, seniors can experience greater vitality, resilience, and joy in their lives, empowering them to age with grace, dignity, and purpose.

CHAPTER TWO

2.1 THE FOUNDATIONS OF CHAIR YOGA

Chair yoga provides a welcoming entry point into the world of yoga, offering a gentle and accessible approach to practicing mindfulness, movement, and relaxation. In this chapter, we'll explore the foundational elements of chair yoga, laying the groundwork for a safe, effective, and fulfilling practice.

1. **Understanding the Chair**: The chair serves as the cornerstone of chair yoga practice, providing stability, support, and accessibility for individuals of all ages and abilities. Before diving into the poses and sequences, it's essential to familiarize yourself with your chair and ensure that it is sturdy, comfortable, and free from obstacles.

2. **Breath Awareness**: Breath is the life force that animates our bodies and calms our minds. In chair yoga, we cultivate awareness of the breath as a means of grounding ourselves in the present moment and connecting with our inner wisdom. Through gentle breathing exercises and mindful awareness, we learn to harness the power of the breath to reduce stress, increase vitality, and promote relaxation.

3. **Mindful Movement**: Chair yoga invites us to move with intention and awareness, honoring the unique capabilities and limitations of our bodies. From gentle stretches to dynamic flows, each movement is performed with mindfulness and presence, allowing us to explore the full range of motion while respecting our individual needs and boundaries.

4. **Modifications and Props**: One of the key principles of chair yoga is adaptability. Everybody is different, and chair yoga offers a variety of modifications and props to accommodate diverse needs and abilities. Whether using blocks, straps, or bolsters to support a pose, or making adjustments to suit your comfort level, it's important to listen to your body and practice with compassion and self-awareness.

5. **Safety First**: As with any form of exercise, safety is paramount in chair yoga. It's essential to practice mindfully, paying attention to any sensations of discomfort or strain and adjusting accordingly. If you have any pre-existing health conditions or concerns, it's advisable to consult with a healthcare professional before beginning a new exercise program.

By laying a strong foundation in the principles of chair yoga, we create a solid framework for a sustainable and transformative practice. In the chapters that follow, we'll explore specific poses, sequences, and techniques designed to enhance flexibility, strength, balance, and well-being, empowering you to cultivate greater vitality and joy in your life through the practice of chair yoga.

2.2 Exploring the Basics: Detailed Explanation of Chair Yoga Poses, Modifications, and Props

Chair yoga offers a rich tapestry of poses, modifications, and props that cater to individuals of all ages, abilities, and physical conditions. In this section, we'll dive into the fundamental aspects of chair yoga, providing a comprehensive guide to help you explore the diverse range of poses and adapt them to suit your unique needs and preferences.

1. **Seated Poses**: Seated poses form the foundation of chair yoga, allowing practitioners to cultivate strength, flexibility, and mindfulness from the comfort of their chairs. Examples of seated poses include:

    - Seated Mountain Pose: Sit tall with feet flat on the floor, grounding down through the sit bones while lengthening the spine and reaching the arms overhead.

    - Seated Forward Fold: From a seated position, hinge at the hips to fold forward, allowing the chest to rest on the thighs and the arms to dangle towards the floor.

    - Seated Twist: Sit tall and gently rotate the torso to one side, placing one hand on the opposite knee and the other hand on the back of the chair for support.

2. **Standing Poses with Chair Support**: While chair yoga is primarily practiced seated, the chair can also be used to provide support in standing poses, offering

stability and balance for individuals who may have difficulty standing unsupported. Examples of standing poses with chair support include:

- Chair Warrior I: Stand behind the chair with hands resting lightly on the back for support, step one foot back into a lunge position, bending the front knee and pressing through the back heel.

- Chair Tree Pose: Stand tall beside the chair, place one hand on the back for support, and bring the sole of one foot to rest on the inner thigh or calf of the standing leg.

3. **Modifications**: Chair yoga embraces the concept of modification, allowing practitioners to adapt poses to suit their individual needs and abilities. Some common modifications include:

    - Using props such as blocks, straps, or blankets to support and enhance poses.

    - Adjusting the range of motion or intensity of a pose to accommodate limitations or discomfort.

    - Utilizing variations of poses to target specific areas of the body or address particular concerns.

4. **Props**: Props are invaluable tools in chair yoga, providing support, stability, and assistance as needed. Some commonly used props include:

- Yoga Blocks: Blocks can be placed under the feet, hands, or sit bones to provide additional height and support in poses.

- Yoga Straps: Straps can be used to extend reach and deepen stretches, particularly for individuals with limited flexibility or range of motion.

- Bolsters or Cushions: Bolsters or cushions can be placed behind the back or under the knees for added comfort and support in seated poses.

By exploring the basics of chair yoga poses, modifications, and props, you'll gain a deeper understanding of how to adapt the practice to suit your unique needs and preferences. Whether you're seeking to enhance flexibility, build strength, or cultivate mindfulness, chair yoga offers a versatile and accessible pathway to greater well-being and vitality.

2.3 Safety First: Tips for Practicing Safely and Effectively in Chair Yoga

Practicing chair yoga is a wonderful way to improve flexibility, strength, and overall well-being, but it's essential to prioritize safety to prevent injuries and ensure a positive experience. In this section, we'll explore key tips for practicing chair yoga safely and effectively, focusing on posture alignment and breathing techniques.

1. **Posture Alignment**:

    - Sit Tall: Maintain an upright and elongated spine throughout your practice. Imagine a string pulling you gently upward from the crown of your head.

    - Engage Core Muscles: Activate your abdominal muscles to support your lower back and stabilize your torso. This helps maintain proper alignment and prevents strain on the spine.

    - Align Hips and Knees: Keep your hips and knees at a 90-degree angle when sitting in the chair, with feet flat on the floor. This helps distribute weight evenly and promotes stability.

    - Relax Shoulders: Soften and relax your shoulders away from your ears. Avoid hunching or tensing the shoulders, which can lead to tension and discomfort.

2. **Breathing Techniques**:
    - Deep Belly Breathing: Practice diaphragmatic breathing by inhaling deeply through your nose, allowing your belly to expand as you fill your lungs with air. Exhale slowly and fully through your mouth, drawing your belly in towards your spine. This type of breathing promotes relaxation and reduces stress.
    - Coordinate Breath with Movement: Sync your breath with your movements to create a flowing and mindful practice. Inhale as you lengthen or expand, and exhale as you contract or release. This rhythmic breathing enhances the mind-body connection and fosters a sense of calm and focus.
    - Maintain a Steady Breath: Avoid holding your breath or breathing shallowly during poses. Keep your breath smooth, steady, and continuous, even if the pose feels challenging. This helps oxygenate your muscles and promotes endurance and relaxation.
3. **Listen to Your Body**:
    - Honor Your Limits: Respect your body's signals and avoid pushing yourself beyond your comfort zone. If a pose feels painful or uncomfortable, ease out of it or modify as needed.

- Modify as Necessary: Use props or modifications to adapt poses to suit your individual needs and abilities. There's no one-size-fits-all approach in yoga, so don't hesitate to make adjustments that feel right for you.

- Take Breaks: If you feel fatigued or overwhelmed during your practice, take a break and rest as needed. Listen to your body's cues and pace yourself accordingly.

4. **Stay Hydrated and Energized**:

    - Drink Water: Stay hydrated by drinking water before, during, and after your practice. Dehydration can contribute to muscle cramps and fatigue, so make sure to replenish fluids regularly.

    - Eat Lightly: Avoid practicing yoga on a full stomach, as this can cause discomfort and interfere with your ability to move and breathe comfortably. Opt for light, nourishing meals or snacks before your practice to maintain energy levels without feeling weighed down.

By prioritizing safety, posture alignment, and mindful breathing techniques in your chair yoga practice, you can enjoy the many benefits of yoga while minimizing the risk of injury and promoting a positive and rewarding experience. Remember to listen to your body, practice with awareness, and approach each session with curiosity and compassion.

2.4 Setting Up Your Space: Guidance on Creating a Comfortable and Conducive Environment for Practice

Creating a supportive environment for your chair yoga practice is essential for enhancing focus, relaxation, and overall well-being. In this section, we'll explore practical tips for setting up your space to ensure comfort, safety, and enjoyment during your practice.

1. **Choose a Quiet and Peaceful Area**:
    - Select a space in your home that is free from distractions and noise. Ideally, choose a quiet room where you can practice without interruption.
    - If possible, create a dedicated yoga space where you can leave your chair set up and ready for practice. This helps establish a sense of ritual and encourages consistency in your practice routine.

2. **Clear the Space**:
    - Clear any clutter or obstacles from the area where you'll be practicing. This creates a safe and spacious environment for movement and reduces the risk of tripping or bumping into objects.
    - If practicing in a shared space, communicate with family members or roommates to ensure they are aware of your practice time and can respect your need for uninterrupted space.

3. **Set the Mood**:

- Create a calming atmosphere by dimming the lights or lighting candles or incense. Soft, ambient lighting can help promote relaxation and focus during your practice.

- Play soothing music or nature sounds to enhance the sensory experience and create a tranquil ambiance. Choose music that complements your practice and helps you connect with your breath and body.

4. **Gather Props and Equipment**:

    - Gather any props or equipment you may need for your practice, such as yoga blocks, straps, or cushions. Place them within easy reach so you can access them as needed during your practice.

    - If you're using a chair with wheels, consider securing it in place with a non-slip mat or by placing it against a wall to prevent it from moving during poses.

5. **Ensure Comfort**:

    - Choose a comfortable and supportive chair that allows you to sit with feet flat on the floor and knees at a 90-degree angle. Avoid chairs with arms that restrict movement or cause discomfort.

    - Use cushions or blankets to enhance comfort and support during seated poses. Place a cushion behind your lower back for added support and comfort, or use a folded blanket to cushion your seat.

6. **Mindful Arrangement**:
    - Arrange your props and equipment mindfully, keeping them organized and aesthetically pleasing. A tidy and harmonious space can enhance your sense of well-being and make it easier to focus on your practice.
    - Consider incorporating elements of nature, such as plants or natural materials, into your space to create a sense of connection with the natural world and promote a feeling of grounding and serenity.

By taking the time to set up your space thoughtfully and intentionally, you can create a nurturing environment that supports and enhances your chair yoga practice. Whether you're practicing alone or with others, cultivating a comfortable and conducive space allows you to immerse yourself fully in the present moment and reap the full benefits of your practice.

CHAPTER THREE

3.1 CHAIR YOGA FOR MOBILITY AND FLEXIBILITY

Chair yoga offers a gentle yet effective approach to improving mobility and flexibility, making it an ideal practice for individuals of all ages and abilities, including seniors. In this section, we'll explore how chair yoga can enhance range of motion, loosen stiff joints, and promote greater flexibility throughout the body.

1. **Gentle Warm-Ups**:
    - Chair yoga sessions often begin with gentle warm-up exercises to prepare the body for movement and reduce the risk of injury. These may include gentle neck rolls, shoulder shrugs, and wrist circles to loosen up tight muscles and joints.
    - Warm-up movements are performed slowly and mindfully, allowing participants to connect with their breath and gently awaken the body without strain or discomfort.

2. **Dynamic Stretching**:
    - Chair yoga incorporates a variety of dynamic stretching exercises to improve flexibility and range of motion. Dynamic stretches involve moving the body through a full range of motion while maintaining control and awareness.
    - Examples of dynamic stretches in chair yoga include arm circles, leg swings, and spinal

twists, which help to increase blood flow, lubricate the joints, and release tension in the muscles.

3. **Joint Mobility Exercises**:
   - Chair yoga includes specific exercises designed to improve mobility in key joints such as the shoulders, hips, and spine. These exercises focus on moving the joints through their natural range of motion to maintain or restore flexibility and function.
   - Joint mobility exercises may involve gentle rotations, circles, or figure-eight movements performed with awareness and control to prevent strain or injury.

4. **Targeted Stretches**:
   - Chair yoga offers a variety of seated and standing stretches to target specific areas of the body and address common areas of stiffness or tightness. These stretches can be modified to suit individual needs and abilities.
   - Examples of targeted stretches in chair yoga include seated forward folds to stretch the hamstrings and lower back, seated spinal twists to increase mobility in the spine, and standing quad stretches to release tension in the front of the thighs.

5. **Breath Awareness**:
   - Breath awareness is an integral part of chair yoga for mobility and flexibility.

Practitioners are encouraged to synchronize their breath with movement, using the breath as a tool to deepen stretches, increase relaxation, and enhance body awareness.

- By connecting breath with movement, participants can release tension more effectively and access deeper levels of flexibility without force or strain.

6. **Progressive Approach**:

    - Chair yoga takes a progressive approach to improving mobility and flexibility, gradually increasing the intensity and duration of stretches over time. Participants are encouraged to listen to their bodies and work within their comfort zone to avoid overstretching or pushing too hard.

    - Consistent practice over time can lead to noticeable improvements in mobility and flexibility, allowing individuals to move more freely and comfortably in their daily lives.

Chair yoga for mobility and flexibility offers a gentle yet powerful way to improve range of motion, release tension, and enhance overall well-being. By incorporating dynamic stretching, joint mobility exercises, targeted stretches, and breath awareness into your practice, you can cultivate greater flexibility and mobility throughout your body, promoting a sense of vitality and ease in your movements.

3.2 Gentle Warm-Ups: Sequences Focusing on Loosening Stiff Joints and Improving Flexibility

Gentle warm-up sequences are essential in chair yoga as they help prepare the body for movement, increase circulation, and reduce the risk of injury. These sequences focus on loosening stiff joints and improving flexibility in a safe and effective manner. Below are some examples of gentle warm-up sequences commonly used in chair yoga:

1. **Neck Rolls**:
    - Sit comfortably in your chair with your feet flat on the floor and your spine tall.
    - Inhale as you gently drop your chin towards your chest, feeling a stretch along the back of your neck.
    - Exhale as you slowly roll your head to the right, bringing your right ear towards your right shoulder. Hold for a breath.
    - Inhale as you return your head to center, then exhale as you roll your head to the left, bringing your left ear towards your left shoulder. Hold for a breath.
    - Continue this gentle rolling motion from side to side for several breaths, allowing your neck muscles to relax and release tension.

2. **Shoulder Shrugs**:
    - Sit tall in your chair with your arms relaxed at your sides.

- Inhale as you shrug your shoulders up towards your ears, lifting them as high as you can without strain.
- Exhale as you gently release your shoulders down, allowing them to relax and soften.
- Repeat this shrugging motion several times, synchronizing your breath with the movement to create a sense of fluidity and ease in your shoulders.

3. **Wrist Circles**:
   - Extend your arms out in front of you with your palms facing down.
   - Inhale as you rotate your wrists in a clockwise direction, circling your hands several times.
   - Exhale as you reverse the direction of the circles, rotating your wrists in a counterclockwise direction.
   - Continue this gentle wrist circling motion, focusing on creating smooth and fluid movements to increase mobility and flexibility in your wrists and forearms.

4. **Ankle Circles**:
   - Sit with your feet flat on the floor and your knees aligned with your hips.
   - Inhale as you lift your right foot off the floor, flexing your toes towards your shin.

- Exhale as you rotate your right ankle in a clockwise direction, circling your foot several times.
- Inhale as you reverse the direction of the circles, rotating your ankle in a counterclockwise direction.
- Repeat this ankle circling motion on your left foot, focusing on creating space and mobility in your ankle joints.

5. **Spinal Twists**:
    - Sit tall in your chair with your feet planted firmly on the floor.
    - Inhale as you lengthen your spine and lift your arms overhead.
    - Exhale as you twist gently to the right, placing your left hand on the outside of your right knee and your right hand on the back of the chair for support.
    - Inhale to lengthen through your spine, and exhale to deepen the twist, gently rotating your torso to the right.
    - Hold the twist for a few breaths, then inhale to return to center and repeat on the other side.

These gentle warm-up sequences are designed to increase circulation, promote flexibility, and prepare the body for deeper stretches and movements in chair yoga practice. By incorporating these sequences into your routine, you can help alleviate stiffness, improve joint mobility, and enhance overall well-being in a safe and mindful manner.

3.3 Mobility Boosters: Exercises to Enhance Range of Motion and Ease Everyday Movements

Maintaining and improving mobility is essential for performing daily tasks with ease and reducing the risk of injury as we age. Chair yoga offers a variety of exercises specifically designed to enhance range of motion in joints and muscles, promoting greater mobility and flexibility. Let's explore some mobility boosters that can help you move more freely and comfortably in your daily life:

1. **Seated Cat-Cow Stretch**:
    - Sit comfortably in your chair with your feet flat on the floor and your hands resting on your thighs.
    - Inhale as you arch your back, lifting your chest and gently tilting your pelvis forward (Cow Pose).
    - Exhale as you round your spine, tucking your chin towards your chest and drawing your belly button towards your spine (Cat Pose).
    - Continue flowing between Cat and Cow Pose with your breath, moving slowly and mindfully to increase flexibility in your spine and improve posture.

2. **Knee Lifts**:
    - Sit tall in your chair with your feet flat on the floor and your hands resting on the armrests or thighs for support.
    - Inhale as you lift your right knee towards your chest, bringing it as close to your body as comfortable.

- Exhale as you gently lower your right foot back to the floor.
- Repeat on the left side, lifting and lowering your left knee with each breath.
- Continue alternating between right and left knee lifts, moving at your own pace and focusing on maintaining stability and balance.

3. **Hip Circles**:
   - Sit towards the front edge of your chair with your feet planted firmly on the floor and your hands resting on your thighs.
   - Inhale as you lift your right knee towards your chest, then exhale as you rotate your knee out to the side, drawing circles with your knee.
   - Inhale to reverse the direction of the circles, bringing your knee back to center and then circling it in the opposite direction.
   - Repeat the hip circles on the left side, moving slowly and smoothly to increase mobility and flexibility in your hip joints.

4. **Shoulder Rolls**:
   - Sit tall with your feet flat on the floor and your hands resting on your thighs or the armrests of your chair.
   - Inhale as you lift your shoulders up towards your ears, then exhale as you roll them back

and down, squeezing your shoulder blades together.

- Inhale to roll your shoulders forward and up towards your ears, then exhale as you roll them back and down again.
- Continue this rolling motion, syncing your breath with the movement to release tension and increase mobility in your shoulder joints.

5. **Seated Forward Fold**:
    - Sit towards the front edge of your chair with your feet hip-width apart and your spine tall.
    - Inhale as you lengthen through your spine, then exhale as you hinge forward from your hips, folding your torso over your thighs.
    - Allow your arms to hang loosely towards the floor, or reach for your shins or feet if comfortable.
    - Hold the forward fold for a few breaths, feeling a gentle stretch along the back of your legs and spine.
    - Inhale to slowly rise back up to a seated position, stacking your vertebrae one by one.

Incorporating these mobility boosters into your daily routine can help increase flexibility, improve joint mobility, and ease everyday movements. Practice them regularly with mindfulness and awareness, moving slowly and gently to avoid strain or discomfort. Over time, you'll notice improvements in your mobility, making it easier to move with grace and ease in your daily life.

3.4 Targeted Stretches: Techniques for Specific Areas like Hips, Shoulders, and Spine

Targeted stretches in chair yoga focus on specific areas of the body to release tension, improve flexibility, and enhance mobility. By addressing key areas such as the hips, shoulders, and spine, these stretches help alleviate stiffness and discomfort while promoting a greater sense of ease and well-being. Let's explore techniques for targeted stretches in each of these areas:

1. **Hip Opener Stretch**:
   - Sit tall in your chair with your feet flat on the floor and your hands resting on your thighs.
   - Cross your right ankle over your left knee, creating a figure-four shape with your legs.
   - Inhale as you lengthen through your spine, then exhale as you gently press down on your right knee, feeling a stretch in your right hip and outer thigh.
   - Hold the stretch for several breaths, then release and switch sides, crossing your left ankle over your right knee and repeating the stretch on the opposite side.

2. **Shoulder Stretch**:
   - Sit tall with your feet flat on the floor and your hands resting on your thighs.
   - Inhale as you reach your right arm up towards the ceiling, then exhale as you bend your elbow and reach your right hand down your back.

- Reach your left hand behind your back and try to clasp your fingertips together, allowing your shoulders to open and stretch.
- Hold the stretch for a few breaths, feeling a gentle opening across the front of your right shoulder.
- Release and switch sides, repeating the stretch with your left arm reaching up and your right hand reaching down your back.

3. **Seated Spinal Twist**:
   - Sit tall in your chair with your feet flat on the floor and your hands resting on your thighs.
   - Inhale as you lengthen through your spine, then exhale as you twist gently to the right, placing your left hand on the outside of your right knee and your right hand on the back of the chair for support.
   - Inhale to lengthen through your spine, then exhale to deepen the twist, rotating your torso to the right and gazing over your right shoulder.
   - Hold the twist for several breaths, feeling a gentle stretch along the muscles of your spine and torso.
   - Release and switch sides, twisting to the left and repeating the stretch on the opposite side.

4. **Neck and Shoulder Release**:
   - Sit tall in your chair with your feet flat on the floor and your hands resting on your thighs.

- Inhale as you lengthen through your spine, then exhale as you drop your right ear towards your right shoulder, feeling a stretch along the left side of your neck.
- Hold the stretch for a few breaths, then inhale to return to center and exhale as you repeat the stretch on the opposite side, dropping your left ear towards your left shoulder.
- Continue alternating between right and left side neck stretches, moving slowly and gently to release tension in the neck and shoulders.

By incorporating these targeted stretches into your chair yoga practice, you can release tension, improve flexibility, and enhance mobility in specific areas of the body. Practice with mindfulness and awareness, listening to your body and respecting its limits to avoid strain or discomfort. Over time, you'll experience increased freedom of movement and a greater sense of ease and well-being in your body.

CHAPTER FOUR

4.1 CHAIR YOGA FOR STRENGTH AND BALANCE

Chair yoga offers a unique and accessible approach to building strength and improving balance, making it an ideal practice for individuals of all ages and abilities, including seniors. By incorporating gentle movements, resistance exercises, and stability challenges, chair yoga helps strengthen muscles, improve coordination, and enhance stability, promoting greater independence and confidence in daily activities. Let's explore how chair yoga can be used to cultivate strength and balance:

1. **Strength-Building Poses**:
    - **Chair Pose**: Sit tall in your chair with your feet hip-width apart. Inhale as you raise your arms overhead, palms facing each other. Exhale as you bend your knees and lower your hips towards the chair, as if you were sitting back into a chair. Hold the pose for a few breaths, engaging your thigh muscles and core to support your body weight.
    - **Warrior II Pose**: Sit towards the front edge of your chair with your feet wide apart. Inhale as you extend your arms out to the sides at shoulder height. Exhale as you turn your right foot out to the side and bend your right knee, aligning it with your ankle. Hold the pose for a few breaths, feeling a deep stretch in your inner thighs and strength in your legs. Repeat on the other side.

2. **Resistance Exercises**:
    - **Seated Leg Lifts**: Sit tall in your chair with your feet flat on the floor. Inhale as you extend your right leg out in front of you, keeping it parallel to the floor. Exhale as you lower your leg back down. Repeat on the other side, alternating legs for several repetitions. This exercise strengthens the quadriceps and improves leg strength.
    - **Seated Row**: Sit tall with a resistance band wrapped around the bottoms of your feet. Hold the ends of the band in each hand with palms facing each other. Inhale as you pull the band towards your chest, squeezing your shoulder blades together. Exhale as you release back to starting position. Repeat for several repetitions to strengthen the muscles of the upper back and shoulders.
3. **Balance Challenges**:
    - **Single Leg Balance**: Sit tall with your feet flat on the floor. Inhale as you lift your right foot off the floor, bringing your knee towards your chest. Hold for a few breaths, finding your balance. Exhale as you lower your foot back to the floor. Repeat on the other side, alternating legs for several repetitions to improve balance and stability.
    - **Tree Pose Variation**: Sit tall with your feet flat on the floor. Inhale as you lift your right foot off the floor, placing the sole of your right foot against the inner calf or thigh of

your left leg. Find a focal point to help you balance. Hold for a few breaths, then exhale as you release and repeat on the other side. This pose challenges balance and strengthens the muscles of the standing leg.

4. **Core Strengthening**:

- **Seated Twist with Core Engagement**: Sit tall in your chair with your feet flat on the floor. Inhale as you lengthen through your spine, then exhale as you twist gently to the right, placing your left hand on the outside of your right knee and your right hand on the back of the chair for support. Engage your core muscles as you twist, feeling the muscles of your abdomen working to support the movement. Hold for a few breaths, then inhale to return to center and repeat on the other side.

By incorporating strength-building poses, resistance exercises, balance challenges, and core strengthening techniques into your chair yoga practice, you can improve muscle tone, enhance stability, and increase confidence in your body's ability to move with ease and grace. Practice regularly and with mindfulness, listening to your body and respecting its limits to avoid strain or injury. Over time, you'll experience increased strength, improved balance, and a greater sense of vitality and well-being in your daily life.

4.2 Building Strength: Chair-Based Exercises to Improve Muscle Tone and Stability

Chair-based strength exercises are a valuable component of chair yoga, offering a safe and effective way to improve muscle tone, enhance stability, and increase overall strength. These exercises utilize the support of a chair to provide stability and balance while targeting various muscle groups throughout the body. Let's explore some chair-based strength exercises that you can incorporate into your chair yoga practice:

1. **Seated Squats**:
    - Sit tall in your chair with your feet hip-width apart and your hands resting on your thighs.
    - Inhale as you engage your core and lift your chest, lengthening through your spine.
    - Exhale as you slowly lower your hips towards the chair, bending your knees and keeping your weight in your heels.
    - Pause briefly when your hips are hovering just above the chair, then inhale as you press through your heels to rise back up to standing.
    - Repeat for several repetitions, focusing on maintaining good posture and engaging your leg muscles throughout the movement.

2. **Chair Dips**:
    - Sit towards the front edge of your chair with your hands gripping the front edge of the seat, fingers pointing towards your body.

- Inhale as you engage your core and lift your hips off the chair, using your arms to support your body weight.
- Exhale as you bend your elbows, lowering your hips towards the floor while keeping your back close to the chair.
- Pause briefly when your elbows reach a 90-degree angle, then inhale as you press through your palms to straighten your arms and lift your hips back up.
- Repeat for several repetitions, focusing on maintaining stability in your shoulders and engaging your triceps and chest muscles.

3. **Seated Leg Extensions**:
   - Sit tall in your chair with your feet flat on the floor and your hands resting on your thighs.
   - Inhale as you extend your right leg out in front of you, keeping it parallel to the floor.
   - Exhale as you engage your quadriceps muscles and hold the leg extension for a few breaths.
   - Inhale to bend your knee and lower your foot back to the floor, then repeat on the other side.
   - Continue alternating leg extensions for several repetitions, focusing on maintaining stability in your core and pelvis.

4. **Chair Push-Ups**:
    - Sit towards the front edge of your chair with your hands gripping the sides of the seat, fingers pointing forward.
    - Inhale as you engage your core and lean forward slightly, shifting your weight onto your hands.
    - Exhale as you bend your elbows, lowering your chest towards the seat of the chair while keeping your body in a straight line.
    - Pause briefly when your chest is just above the seat, then inhale as you press through your palms to straighten your arms and lift your chest back up.
    - Repeat for several repetitions, focusing on maintaining stability in your core and shoulders and engaging your chest and arm muscles.

5. **Seated Row**:
    - Sit tall in your chair with your feet flat on the floor and a resistance band wrapped around the bottoms of your feet.
    - Hold the ends of the band in each hand with palms facing each other, arms extended straight out in front of you.
    - Inhale as you pull the band towards your chest, squeezing your shoulder blades together and engaging your upper back muscles.

- Exhale as you slowly release the band back to starting position, maintaining control throughout the movement.
- Repeat for several repetitions, focusing on maintaining good posture and engaging your back and arm muscles.

Incorporate these chair-based strength exercises into your chair yoga practice regularly to improve muscle tone, enhance stability, and increase overall strength. Practice with mindfulness and awareness, focusing on proper form and alignment to maximize the benefits of each exercise. As you gradually build strength and stability, you'll experience increased confidence and vitality in your daily life.

4.3 Finding Balance: Practices to Enhance Equilibrium and Reduce the Risk of Falls

Maintaining balance is essential for mobility, stability, and overall well-being, especially as we age. Chair yoga offers a range of practices designed to enhance equilibrium, improve proprioception, and reduce the risk of falls. These practices focus on strengthening key muscles, refining coordination, and increasing body awareness to promote greater stability and confidence in everyday movements. Let's explore some chair yoga practices to help you find balance:

1. **Seated Mountain Pose**:
    - Sit tall in your chair with your feet flat on the floor and your hands resting on your thighs.
    - Inhale as you lengthen through your spine, lifting your chest and reaching the crown of your head towards the ceiling.

- Exhale as you ground down through your sit bones, feeling a sense of stability and support from the chair beneath you.
- Hold the pose for several breaths, focusing on finding a strong and stable foundation while maintaining ease and relaxation in your body.

2. **One-Leg Balance**:
    - Sit towards the front edge of your chair with your feet flat on the floor and your hands resting on your thighs.
    - Inhale as you lift your right foot off the floor, bringing your knee towards your chest.
    - Exhale as you hold the position, finding your balance and stability.
    - Hold for a few breaths, then inhale to lower your right foot back to the floor.
    - Repeat on the other side, lifting your left foot off the floor and holding for a few breaths before lowering it back down.

3. **Chair Warrior III**:
    - Sit towards the front edge of your chair with your feet hip-width apart and your hands resting on your thighs.
    - Inhale as you lift your right foot off the floor, extending it straight back behind you.
    - Exhale as you hinge forward from your hips, bringing your torso parallel to the floor and reaching your arms forward.

- Hold the pose for several breaths, finding a strong and stable line of energy from your fingertips to your heel.
- Inhale to return to a seated position, then repeat on the other side, lifting your left foot off the floor and extending it straight back behind you.

4. **Seated Tree Pose**:
   - Sit tall in your chair with your feet flat on the floor and your hands resting on your thighs.
   - Inhale as you lift your right foot off the floor, placing the sole of your right foot against the inner calf or thigh of your left leg.
   - Exhale as you press your foot into your leg and your leg into your foot, finding stability and support in the pose.
   - Hold for several breaths, finding a focal point to help you maintain balance and focus.
   - Inhale to release and lower your right foot back to the floor, then repeat on the other side.

5. **Mindful Walking**:
   - Stand behind your chair with your feet hip-width apart and your hands resting lightly on the back of the chair for support.
   - Inhale as you lift your right heel off the floor, transferring your weight onto the ball of your right foot.

- Exhale as you slowly lower your right heel back to the floor, feeling the connection with the ground beneath you.
- Repeat on the left side, lifting and lowering your left heel with each breath.
- Continue this mindful walking practice, moving slowly and deliberately, and paying attention to the sensations in your feet and legs as you shift your weight.

Incorporate these practices into your chair yoga routine regularly to enhance equilibrium, improve balance, and reduce the risk of falls. Practice with mindfulness and awareness, focusing on maintaining stability and ease in your body while exploring your edge. Over time, you'll experience greater confidence and steadiness in your movements, allowing you to navigate daily activities with grace and poise.

4.4 Core Connection: Strengthening the Core Muscles for Better Posture and Stability

A strong core is essential for maintaining proper posture, stability, and overall physical well-being. In chair yoga, focusing on strengthening the core muscles can significantly improve balance, support the spine, and enhance overall stability. By incorporating targeted exercises that engage the core muscles, you can cultivate greater strength and resilience in the center of your body. Let's explore some chair yoga practices to help you establish a strong core connection:

1. **Seated Cat-Cow Pose**:
    - Sit tall in your chair with your feet flat on the floor and your hands resting on your thighs.
    - Inhale as you arch your back, lifting your chest and gently tilting your pelvis forward (Cow Pose).
    - Exhale as you round your spine, tucking your chin towards your chest and drawing your belly button towards your spine (Cat Pose).
    - Flow between Cat and Cow Pose with your breath, engaging your core muscles to support the movement and maintain stability in your spine.
2. **Seated Spinal Twist with Core Engagement**:
    - Sit tall in your chair with your feet flat on the floor and your hands resting on your thighs.
    - Inhale as you lengthen through your spine, then exhale as you twist gently to the right, placing your left hand on the outside of your

right knee and your right hand on the back of the chair for support.

- Engage your core muscles as you twist, feeling the muscles of your abdomen working to support the movement.
- Hold the twist for several breaths, then inhale to return to center and repeat on the other side.

3. **Seated Boat Pose**:
    - Sit towards the front edge of your chair with your feet flat on the floor and your hands resting lightly on the sides of the chair for support.
    - Inhale as you lift your legs off the floor, bringing your knees towards your chest and balancing on your sit bones.
    - Extend your arms forward at shoulder height, palms facing each other, and engage your core muscles to maintain balance.
    - Hold the pose for several breaths, feeling the strength and stability in your core, then exhale as you lower your feet back to the floor.

4. **Seated Side Bend**:
    - Sit tall in your chair with your feet flat on the floor and your hands resting on your thighs.
    - Inhale as you reach your right arm overhead, lengthening through your side body.

- Exhale as you side bend to the left, sliding your left hand down your left thigh and stretching through the right side of your body.
- Engage your core muscles to support the side bend and maintain stability in your spine.
- Hold the stretch for several breaths, then inhale to return to center and repeat on the other side.

5. **Seated Knee-to-Elbow Crunch**:
   - Sit tall in your chair with your feet flat on the floor and your hands resting lightly on the sides of the chair for support.
   - Inhale as you lift your right knee towards your chest, bringing it as close to your right elbow as possible.
   - Exhale as you engage your core muscles and draw your knee and elbow towards each other, feeling the contraction in your abdominal muscles.
   - Hold the crunch for a moment, then inhale to release and extend your leg back to starting position.
   - Repeat on the other side, lifting your left knee towards your left elbow and performing the crunch with control.

Incorporate these core-strengthening exercises into your chair yoga practice regularly to improve posture, enhance stability, and cultivate a strong connection to your center. Practice with mindfulness and awareness, focusing on engaging the core muscles with each movement to maximize the benefits. As you gradually build strength in your core, you'll experience improved posture, increased stability, and greater overall vitality in your daily life.

CHAPTER FIVE

5.1 CHAIR YOGA FOR MIND-BODY CONNECTION

Chair yoga offers a unique opportunity to cultivate a deep mind-body connection, fostering harmony and balance within oneself. Through gentle movements, breath awareness, and mindfulness practices, chair yoga encourages individuals to explore the interplay between the physical body, breath, and mind, promoting a sense of inner calm and well-being. Let's delve into some key aspects of chair yoga for nurturing the mind-body connection:

1. **Breath Awareness**:
    - Chair yoga emphasizes the importance of breath awareness as a foundation for cultivating mindfulness and presence. Practitioners are encouraged to connect with their breath, observing its rhythm and quality as they move through various poses and exercises.
    - Breath awareness techniques, such as deep belly breathing and conscious breathing, help to calm the nervous system, reduce stress, and enhance overall relaxation. By synchronizing movement with breath, individuals can deepen their mind-body connection and experience a greater sense of inner peace.

2. **Mindful Movement**:
    - Chair yoga encourages mindful movement, inviting practitioners to move with intention

and awareness. Each movement is performed slowly and deliberately, allowing individuals to fully experience the sensations in their body and cultivate a sense of presence.

- By bringing mindful attention to the present moment, individuals can deepen their mind-body connection and develop a greater appreciation for the body's abilities and limitations. Mindful movement practices help to increase body awareness, improve proprioception, and enhance overall coordination and balance.

3. **Body Scan Meditation**:
    - Chair yoga often incorporates body scan meditation, a mindfulness practice that involves systematically bringing awareness to different parts of the body. Practitioners are guided to observe sensations, tensions, and areas of ease or discomfort, cultivating a non-judgmental awareness of the body.
    - Body scan meditation promotes relaxation, stress reduction, and greater self-awareness. By tuning into the physical sensations present in the body, individuals can release tension, alleviate pain, and cultivate a deeper sense of connection with themselves.

4. **Visualization**:
    - Visualization techniques are commonly used in chair yoga to enhance the mind-body connection and promote relaxation and healing. Practitioners are guided to visualize

peaceful scenes, calming imagery, or positive affirmations, allowing the mind to focus and quieten.

- Visualization practices can help reduce anxiety, enhance mood, and improve overall well-being. By engaging the power of the imagination, individuals can access a deeper state of relaxation and connection with their inner selves.

5. **Intention Setting**:

    - Chair yoga often begins with setting an intention or a focus for the practice, guiding practitioners to connect with their deeper motivations and aspirations. Intention setting helps to cultivate mindfulness and purpose, anchoring individuals in the present moment and guiding their practice with clarity and intention.

    - By setting a positive intention, individuals can align their actions with their values and goals, fostering a deeper sense of meaning and fulfillment in their yoga practice and in life.

Chair yoga offers a holistic approach to nurturing the mind-body connection, integrating breath awareness, mindful movement, meditation, visualization, and intention setting to promote overall well-being and inner harmony. Through regular practice, individuals can cultivate a deeper sense of self-awareness, resilience, and peace, enriching their lives both on and off the yoga mat.

5.2 The Power of Breath: Deep Breathing Exercises for Relaxation and Stress Relief

Breath is a powerful tool that can profoundly impact our physical, mental, and emotional well-being. In chair yoga, deep breathing exercises are essential for promoting relaxation, reducing stress, and cultivating a sense of calmness and clarity. By harnessing the power of the breath, individuals can tap into their body's natural relaxation response and experience a greater sense of ease and tranquility. Let's explore some deep breathing exercises that you can practice in chair yoga:

1. **Abdominal Breathing**:
    - Sit comfortably in your chair with your feet flat on the floor and your hands resting on your thighs.
    - Close your eyes if comfortable, and take a few natural breaths to settle into the present moment.
    - Place one hand on your abdomen and the other hand on your chest.
    - Inhale deeply through your nose, allowing your abdomen to expand as you fill your lungs with air.
    - Exhale slowly through your mouth, gently drawing your navel towards your spine to expel the breath completely.
    - Continue this deep abdominal breathing for several rounds, focusing on the sensation of the breath moving in and out of your body.

2. **4-7-8 Breath**:
    - Sit comfortably with your feet flat on the floor and your hands resting on your thighs.
    - Close your eyes and take a few natural breaths to center yourself.
    - Inhale deeply through your nose for a count of four seconds, allowing your abdomen to expand.
    - Hold your breath for a count of seven seconds, feeling the fullness of the breath in your lungs.
    - Exhale slowly and completely through your mouth for a count of eight seconds, emptying your lungs completely.
    - Repeat this 4-7-8 breath cycle for several rounds, allowing each breath to soothe and relax your body and mind.

3. **Alternate Nostril Breathing**:
    - Sit comfortably with your feet flat on the floor and your spine tall.
    - Rest your left hand on your left knee and bring your right hand towards your face.
    - Use your right thumb to close your right nostril and inhale deeply through your left nostril.
    - Close your left nostril with your right ring finger, and exhale slowly and completely through your right nostril.

- Inhale deeply through your right nostril, then close it with your right thumb and exhale through your left nostril.
- Continue alternating between inhaling and exhaling through each nostril for several rounds, focusing on the rhythm and flow of your breath.

4. **Ocean Breathing (Ujjayi Breath)**:
    - Sit comfortably with your feet flat on the floor and your hands resting on your thighs.
    - Close your eyes and take a few natural breaths to center yourself.
    - Inhale deeply through your nose, slightly constricting the back of your throat to create a soft "ocean" sound as you breathe in.
    - Exhale slowly and audibly through your nose, maintaining the gentle constriction in the back of your throat.
    - Continue this ujjayi breath for several rounds, allowing the rhythmic sound of your breath to soothe and calm your nervous system.

5. **Square Breathing**:
    - Sit comfortably with your feet flat on the floor and your hands resting on your thighs.
    - Imagine a square shape in your mind, with four equal sides.
    - Inhale deeply through your nose as you count to four, tracing the first side of the square.

- Hold your breath for a count of four as you trace the second side of the square.

- Exhale slowly and completely through your nose for a count of four as you trace the third side of the square.

- Hold your breath for a count of four as you trace the fourth side of the square.

- Repeat this square breath pattern for several rounds, focusing on the steady rhythm and even length of each breath.

These deep breathing exercises are valuable tools for promoting relaxation, reducing stress, and cultivating a greater sense of inner peace and well-being. Incorporate them into your chair yoga practice regularly to harness the power of the breath and experience the transformative effects on your mind, body, and spirit.

5.3 Meditation in Motion: Incorporating Mindfulness into Chair Yoga Poses

Chair yoga offers a beautiful opportunity to cultivate mindfulness in motion, allowing practitioners to bring their full attention and awareness to the present moment while moving through gentle poses and exercises. By integrating mindfulness into chair yoga practice, individuals can deepen their mind-body connection, enhance relaxation, and experience a greater sense of peace and well-being. Let's explore how you can incorporate mindfulness into chair yoga poses:

1. **Body Awareness**:
   - Begin by bringing your attention to the sensations in your body as you sit in your chair. Notice the points of contact between your body and the chair, the feeling of your feet on the ground, and any areas of tension or ease.
   - As you move through chair yoga poses, maintain awareness of the subtle shifts and sensations in your body. Notice how each movement feels, and explore the range of motion with curiosity and openness.
   - By tuning into the sensations in your body, you can deepen your connection to the present moment and cultivate greater body awareness.

2. **Breath Awareness**:
   - Connect your breath with your movement as you flow through chair yoga poses. Pay

attention to the rhythm of your breath, allowing it to guide the pace and timing of your movements.

- Notice the sensations of the breath as it moves in and out of your body. Feel the rise and fall of your chest and abdomen with each inhale and exhale.

- By anchoring your awareness in the breath, you can calm the mind, increase relaxation, and deepen your sense of presence in the moment.

3. **Mindful Transitions**:

    - Focus on the transitions between poses as opportunities to practice mindfulness. Slow down your movements and pay attention to the sensations and movements of your body as you transition from one pose to the next.

    - Notice any tendencies to rush or hurry through transitions, and gently bring your attention back to the present moment. Allow each transition to unfold with ease and awareness.

    - By approaching transitions mindfully, you can cultivate greater mindfulness and presence in your chair yoga practice, enhancing the overall experience.

4. **Sensory Awareness**:

    - Engage your senses as you practice chair yoga poses. Notice the sounds around you, the feeling of the air on your skin, and any sights or smells in your environment.

- Allow your senses to guide your attention inward, deepening your connection to the present moment and enriching your experience of each pose.
- By engaging your senses in this way, you can heighten your awareness and experience of the present moment, fostering a deeper sense of mindfulness and presence.

5. **Gratitude and Intention**:
   - Before beginning your chair yoga practice, take a moment to cultivate a sense of gratitude and set an intention for your practice. Reflect on what you are grateful for in this moment and what you hope to cultivate through your practice.
   - Carry this sense of gratitude and intention with you as you move through chair yoga poses, allowing it to infuse your practice with meaning and purpose.
   - By anchoring your practice in gratitude and intention, you can deepen your mindfulness and connect more fully with yourself and the world around you.

Incorporating mindfulness into chair yoga poses offers a powerful way to deepen your mind-body connection, enhance relaxation, and cultivate a greater sense of presence and well-being. By bringing awareness to your body, breath, transitions, senses, and intentions, you can enrich your chair yoga practice and experience the transformative benefits on and off the mat.

5.4 Restorative Relaxation: Techniques for Deep Relaxation and Rejuvenation

Restorative relaxation practices in chair yoga offer valuable techniques to promote deep relaxation, reduce stress, and rejuvenate the mind, body, and spirit. These gentle and nurturing practices focus on releasing tension, calming the nervous system, and fostering a profound sense of ease and well-being. Let's explore some techniques for restorative relaxation in chair yoga:

1. **Guided Relaxation**:
   - Begin by finding a comfortable seated position in your chair, with your feet flat on the floor and your hands resting comfortably in your lap.
   - Close your eyes if it feels comfortable, or soften your gaze downward.
   - Take a few deep breaths to center yourself and invite relaxation into your body and mind.
   - Guided relaxation involves a facilitator or recording guiding you through a series of visualizations and relaxation prompts to induce a state of deep relaxation.
   - Visualizations may include imagining a peaceful scene, such as a serene beach or a tranquil forest, and focusing on sensory

details to evoke a sense of calmness and tranquility.

- Relaxation prompts may include progressive muscle relaxation, where you systematically tense and release different muscle groups in the body, allowing them to relax fully.

2. **Body Scan Meditation**:
    - Sit comfortably in your chair with your feet flat on the floor and your hands resting on your thighs.
    - Close your eyes and take a few deep breaths to center yourself.
    - Begin by bringing your awareness to the top of your head, and slowly scan down through your body, bringing gentle attention to each area as you move downward.
    - Notice any areas of tension or discomfort, and invite them to soften and release with each breath.
    - Continue scanning down through your body, all the way to your toes, allowing yourself to sink deeper into relaxation with each passing moment.

3. **Breath-Based Relaxation**:
    - Sit comfortably in your chair with your feet flat on the floor and your hands resting on your thighs.
    - Close your eyes and take a few deep breaths to center yourself.

- Focus your attention on your breath, noticing the natural rhythm and flow as you inhale and exhale.
- With each inhale, imagine filling your body with relaxation and peace. With each exhale, imagine releasing any tension or stress that you may be holding onto.
- Allow your breath to become slow, deep, and even, as you continue to relax more fully with each breath.

4. **Restorative Yoga Poses**:
   - Incorporate restorative yoga poses into your chair yoga practice to promote relaxation and rejuvenation.
   - Examples of restorative poses in chair yoga include supported forward fold, where you gently fold forward over a bolster or cushion placed on your lap, allowing your spine to lengthen and your muscles to relax deeply.
   - Another restorative pose is supported reclining twist, where you sit sideways in your chair and gently twist your torso towards the back of the chair, using the chair's back for support. This helps to release tension in the spine and promote relaxation in the body.

5. **Progressive Muscle Relaxation**:
   - Sit comfortably in your chair with your feet flat on the floor and your hands resting on your thighs.

- Close your eyes and take a few deep breaths to center yourself.
- Begin by tensing the muscles in your body, starting with your feet and working your way up to your head. Hold the tension for a few seconds, then release and let go completely.
- Notice the sensation of relaxation that follows each release, and allow yourself to sink deeper into relaxation with each progressive muscle group.

Incorporate these restorative relaxation techniques into your chair yoga practice regularly to promote deep relaxation, reduce stress, and rejuvenate your mind, body, and spirit. Practice with patience and compassion for yourself, allowing yourself to fully surrender and let go into the healing power of relaxation.

CHAPTER SIX

6.1 CHAIR YOGA FOR EVERYDAY WELLNESS

Chair yoga offers accessible and effective techniques for promoting everyday wellness, regardless of age, ability, or fitness level. By integrating gentle movements, breath awareness, and mindfulness practices, chair yoga can enhance physical health, mental clarity, and emotional well-being, making it a valuable tool for cultivating overall wellness in daily life. Let's explore how chair yoga can contribute to everyday wellness:

1. **Physical Health Benefits**:
    - Chair yoga poses and exercises are designed to improve flexibility, strength, balance, and circulation, supporting overall physical health and vitality.
    - Regular practice of chair yoga can help alleviate stiffness, reduce joint pain, and increase mobility, making everyday activities easier and more comfortable.
    - Chair yoga also promotes better posture and spinal alignment, reducing the risk of musculoskeletal issues and enhancing overall physical function.

2. **Mental Clarity and Focus**:
    - Chair yoga incorporates mindfulness practices, such as breath awareness and meditation, to cultivate mental clarity, focus, and concentration.

- By learning to anchor the mind in the present moment, individuals can reduce mental chatter, enhance cognitive function, and improve decision-making skills.
- Chair yoga can also help alleviate stress, anxiety, and mental fatigue, promoting a greater sense of calmness and emotional well-being in everyday life.

3. **Stress Reduction and Relaxation**:
    - The gentle, rhythmic movements of chair yoga, combined with deep breathing exercises, promote relaxation, reduce stress, and induce a state of deep calmness and relaxation.
    - Practicing chair yoga regularly can help individuals unwind from the pressures of daily life, release tension held in the body, and foster a greater sense of inner peace and tranquility.
    - Chair yoga can be particularly beneficial for individuals with busy schedules or high-stress jobs, providing a convenient and accessible way to manage stress and promote relaxation throughout the day.

4. **Improved Energy and Vitality**:
    - Chair yoga stimulates the flow of energy throughout the body, revitalizing the mind, body, and spirit and promoting a sense of vitality and well-being.

- The gentle stretching and movement in chair yoga poses help to release stagnant energy, increase circulation, and invigorate the body's systems, leaving practitioners feeling more energized and alive.
- By incorporating chair yoga into their daily routine, individuals can boost their energy levels, enhance productivity, and approach each day with a renewed sense of vigor and enthusiasm.

5. **Emotional Well-Being and Resilience**:
    - Chair yoga fosters emotional well-being and resilience by promoting self-awareness, self-compassion, and emotional regulation.
    - Through mindfulness practices, individuals learn to observe their thoughts and emotions without judgment, cultivating greater emotional balance and resilience in the face of life's challenges.
    - Chair yoga also encourages self-care and self-nurturing, empowering individuals to prioritize their own well-being and develop a deeper sense of inner strength and resilience.

Incorporating chair yoga into your daily routine can have profound and lasting effects on your overall wellness, from improving physical health and mental clarity to reducing stress and enhancing emotional well-being. Whether you practice for a few minutes each day or incorporate longer sessions into your routine, chair yoga offers a gentle and accessible way to support your well-being and live your best life every day.

6.2 Managing Chronic Conditions: Chair Yoga as a Complementary Therapy for Common Ailments like Arthritis and Osteoporosis

Chair yoga offers a gentle and accessible approach to managing chronic conditions such as arthritis and osteoporosis, providing individuals with valuable tools to alleviate symptoms, improve mobility, and enhance overall well-being. As a complementary therapy, chair yoga can be adapted to accommodate various physical limitations and health concerns, making it an ideal option for individuals seeking relief from the challenges associated with chronic conditions. Let's explore how chair yoga can benefit those managing arthritis and osteoporosis:

1. **Arthritis Management**:
    - Chair yoga offers gentle movements and stretches that can help alleviate joint pain, stiffness, and inflammation associated with arthritis.
    - By incorporating slow and mindful movements, chair yoga helps to improve joint mobility and flexibility, reducing the discomfort and limitations caused by arthritis.
    - Specific chair yoga poses, such as gentle stretches for the fingers, wrists, shoulders, hips, and knees, can target areas commonly affected by arthritis, promoting greater comfort and ease of movement.
    - Additionally, chair yoga practices that emphasize breath awareness and relaxation

techniques can help reduce stress, which is known to exacerbate arthritis symptoms.

2. **Osteoporosis Support**:
    - Chair yoga provides a safe and effective way to strengthen bones, improve balance, and reduce the risk of fractures in individuals with osteoporosis.
    - Weight-bearing chair yoga poses, such as seated squats, leg lifts, and heel raises, help to build bone density and strengthen muscles, which are crucial for supporting healthy bones.
    - Chair yoga also incorporates balance-enhancing exercises and poses, such as seated tree pose and one-leg balance, which can help improve stability and reduce the risk of falls, particularly important for individuals with osteoporosis.
    - Additionally, chair yoga practices that focus on alignment and posture can help individuals with osteoporosis maintain proper spinal alignment and reduce the risk of spinal fractures.

3. **Adaptability and Accessibility**:
    - One of the key benefits of chair yoga is its adaptability and accessibility, making it suitable for individuals of all ages and fitness levels, including those with chronic conditions.

- Chair yoga poses can be modified to accommodate specific needs and limitations, allowing individuals with arthritis or osteoporosis to practice safely and comfortably.
- Props such as blankets, bolsters, and blocks can be used to provide additional support and stability, making it easier for individuals with limited mobility or joint pain to participate in chair yoga practice.
- Furthermore, chair yoga can be practiced in a seated position or with the support of a chair for balance, providing options for individuals who may have difficulty standing or bearing weight on their joints.

4. **Pain Management and Stress Reduction**:
   - Chair yoga incorporates relaxation techniques, deep breathing exercises, and mindfulness practices, which can help individuals manage pain and reduce stress associated with chronic conditions like arthritis and osteoporosis.
   - By cultivating awareness of the breath and the present moment, chair yoga helps individuals develop coping strategies for managing discomfort and promoting relaxation.
   - Regular practice of chair yoga can also improve sleep quality, boost mood, and enhance overall quality of life for individuals managing chronic conditions.

5. **Complementary Therapy Approach**:
    - Chair yoga serves as a complementary therapy that can be integrated with conventional medical treatments and therapies for arthritis and osteoporosis.

    - While chair yoga alone may not cure these conditions, it can significantly improve symptoms, enhance mobility, and contribute to overall well-being when practiced consistently over time.

    - Integrating chair yoga into a comprehensive treatment plan can provide individuals with a holistic approach to managing their health, addressing both physical and emotional aspects of their well-being.

In conclusion, chair yoga serves as a valuable complementary therapy for managing chronic conditions like arthritis and osteoporosis, offering gentle movements, adaptability, and stress-reducing techniques that can alleviate symptoms and improve overall quality of life. By incorporating chair yoga into their routine, individuals can empower themselves to take an active role in managing their health and well-being, fostering a sense of empowerment and resilience in the face of chronic illness.

6.3 Improving Sleep: Relaxation Practices to Promote Better Sleep Quality

Sleep plays a vital role in overall health and well-being, yet many individuals struggle with sleep-related issues such as insomnia, restless sleep, or difficulty falling asleep. Chair yoga offers relaxation practices that can help promote better sleep quality by calming the mind, relaxing the body, and creating a conducive environment for restorative rest. Let's explore some relaxation techniques from chair yoga that can support a good night's sleep:

1. **Deep Breathing Exercises**:
    - Deep breathing exercises are a cornerstone of relaxation in chair yoga. Practicing deep, diaphragmatic breathing can activate the body's relaxation response, calming the nervous system and preparing the body for sleep.
    - One effective deep breathing exercise is the 4-7-8 breath: Inhale deeply through the nose for a count of 4, hold the breath for a count of 7, and exhale slowly through the mouth for a count of 8. Repeat this cycle several times before bedtime to induce a state of relaxation.

2. **Progressive Muscle Relaxation**:
    - Progressive muscle relaxation involves systematically tensing and relaxing different muscle groups in the body to release tension and promote relaxation. This technique can help alleviate physical tension and prepare the body for sleep.

- Begin by tensing the muscles in your feet and toes for a few seconds, then release and relax completely. Move upward through the body, tensing and relaxing each muscle group in turn, from the legs and hips to the shoulders, arms, and neck.

3. **Guided Relaxation**:
    - Guided relaxation involves listening to a recorded meditation or visualization that guides you through a series of relaxation prompts. This can be particularly helpful for quieting the mind and promoting a sense of calm before sleep.
    - Look for guided relaxation recordings specifically designed to promote sleep. These may include visualizations of peaceful landscapes, soothing music, or calming affirmations that help create a relaxing atmosphere conducive to sleep.

4. **Restorative Yoga Poses**:
    - Restorative yoga poses can be adapted for a seated or reclined position in a chair, making them accessible for individuals who may have difficulty getting onto the floor. These gentle poses help release tension in the body and promote relaxation.
    - Examples of restorative chair yoga poses that can promote better sleep include seated forward folds, gentle twists, and supported reclining poses using bolsters or cushions for added comfort and support.

5. **Mindfulness Meditation**:
    - Mindfulness meditation involves bringing non-judgmental awareness to the present moment, including sensations in the body, thoughts, and emotions. Practicing mindfulness meditation before bed can help quiet the mind and prepare for sleep.
    - Sit comfortably in a chair with your feet flat on the floor and your hands resting in your lap. Close your eyes and focus on the sensation of your breath as it enters and leaves your body. When thoughts arise, simply acknowledge them without judgment and gently return your focus to the breath.
6. **Creating a Relaxing Bedtime Routine**:
    - In addition to specific relaxation techniques, establishing a relaxing bedtime routine can signal to your body that it's time to wind down and prepare for sleep.
    - Incorporate activities such as gentle stretching, reading, taking a warm bath, or listening to calming music into your bedtime routine. Avoid stimulating activities such as screen time or intense exercise close to bedtime, as these can interfere with sleep.

By incorporating these relaxation practices into your bedtime routine, you can create a calming environment that promotes better sleep quality and overall well-being. Consistency is key, so aim to practice these techniques regularly to reap the full benefits of chair yoga for improved sleep.

6.4 Enhancing Mental Clarity: Techniques for Sharpening Focus and Cognitive Function

In chair yoga, there are specific techniques tailored to enhance mental clarity, sharpen focus, and boost cognitive function. These techniques integrate mindful movement, breathwork, and mindfulness practices to cultivate a sharper mind and improve overall cognitive performance. Let's delve into these techniques with specific examples:

1. **Focused Breathing**:
   - Technique: Practice focused breathing exercises to anchor attention and calm the mind. One such technique is Box Breathing, where you inhale for a count of four, hold for a count of four, exhale for a count of four, and hold for a count of four, repeating the cycle.
   - Example: Sit comfortably in your chair, close your eyes, and bring your awareness to your breath. Inhale deeply through your nose for a count of four, feeling the breath fill your lungs. Hold your breath for a count of four, then exhale slowly through your mouth for a count of four. Hold the breath out for a count of four before repeating the cycle.

2. **Mindful Movement**:
   - Technique: Engage in mindful movement by synchronizing breath with movement, fostering a deep connection between body and mind. Focus on the sensations of each movement to sharpen awareness and concentration.

- Example: Practice Seated Cat-Cow Stretch by inhaling as you arch your back, lifting your chest and rolling your shoulders back (Cow Pose), then exhaling as you round your spine, tucking your chin to your chest (Cat Pose). Coordinate each movement with a slow, deliberate breath to enhance focus and clarity.

3. **Mindfulness Meditation**:
    - Technique: Incorporate mindfulness meditation to train attention and reduce mental clutter. Focus on observing thoughts, sensations, and emotions without judgment, cultivating present-moment awareness.
    - Example: Sit comfortably in your chair with your feet grounded and hands resting on your thighs. Close your eyes and bring your attention to your breath. Notice the sensations of each inhale and exhale, observing thoughts as they arise without getting caught up in them. Return your focus to the breath whenever the mind wanders.

4. **Brain-Boosting Poses**:
    - Technique: Practice chair yoga poses that stimulate circulation to the brain, improving oxygenation and cognitive function. Poses like Seated Forward Fold and Seated Spinal Twist can help release tension in the spine and increase blood flow to the brain.
    - Example: In Seated Forward Fold, sit on the edge of your chair with feet hip-width apart.

Inhale, lengthen your spine, then exhale, hinge at the hips, and fold forward, resting your hands on the floor or grabbing hold of your shins. Hold for a few breaths, feeling the stretch in your spine and the release of tension in your neck and shoulders.

5. **Visualization**:

    - Technique: Utilize visualization techniques to enhance mental clarity and focus. Imagine a calming scene or visualize yourself successfully completing a task to boost motivation and concentration.

    - Example: Close your eyes and imagine yourself sitting in a peaceful garden surrounded by lush greenery and blooming flowers. Engage your senses by visualizing the vibrant colors, feeling the warmth of the sun on your skin, and hearing the gentle rustle of leaves in the breeze. Allow this visualization to bring a sense of calm and clarity to your mind.

By incorporating these specific techniques into your chair yoga practice, you can sharpen your focus, enhance cognitive function, and cultivate a clearer and more alert mind. Consistent practice of these techniques can lead to improved mental clarity, increased productivity, and greater overall well-being.

CHAPTER SEVEN

7.1 CHAIR YOGA FOR LIFE ENRICHMENT

Chair yoga is not just a physical practice; it's a holistic approach to well-being that can enrich every aspect of life. Beyond its benefits for the body, chair yoga offers valuable tools and techniques for enhancing mental, emotional, and spiritual well-being, ultimately contributing to a more fulfilling and enriched life. Let's explore how chair yoga can enrich your life:

1. **Physical Vitality**:
    - Chair yoga promotes physical vitality by improving flexibility, strength, balance, and mobility. These benefits not only enhance everyday activities but also contribute to a greater sense of energy and vitality.
    - With increased physical vitality, individuals may find themselves more capable and confident in navigating daily tasks and pursuing activities they enjoy, leading to a more active and fulfilling lifestyle.

2. **Emotional Well-Being**:
    - Chair yoga incorporates mindfulness practices, such as breath awareness and meditation, that can help individuals manage stress, anxiety, and other emotional challenges.
    - By learning to cultivate a greater sense of self-awareness and self-compassion, individuals can develop healthier coping mechanisms and a more positive outlook on

life, fostering emotional resilience and well-being.

3. **Mental Clarity and Focus**:
   - Chair yoga techniques for sharpening focus and cognitive function, such as mindful movement and breathwork, can enhance mental clarity and concentration.
   - With improved mental clarity and focus, individuals may experience greater productivity, creativity, and mental agility, enabling them to approach tasks and challenges with clarity and confidence.

4. **Social Connection**:
   - Chair yoga classes provide opportunities for social connection and community building, fostering a sense of belonging and support among participants.
   - Engaging in chair yoga with others can create a supportive environment where individuals can share experiences, build friendships, and cultivate a sense of connection and camaraderie.

5. **Spiritual Growth**:
   - Chair yoga offers a space for spiritual exploration and growth, inviting individuals to connect with their inner selves and explore deeper dimensions of existence.
   - Through practices such as mindfulness meditation, visualization, and reflection, individuals can cultivate a sense of inner

peace, purpose, and meaning, enriching their spiritual lives and deepening their connection to the world around them.

6. **Quality of Life**:
    - Ultimately, chair yoga contributes to a higher quality of life by promoting holistic well-being across physical, emotional, mental, and spiritual dimensions.
    - By integrating chair yoga into their daily routine, individuals can experience greater balance, harmony, and fulfillment in their lives, leading to a more enriched and meaningful existence.

Whether you're looking to improve your physical health, manage stress, enhance your mental clarity, or cultivate a deeper sense of connection and purpose, chair yoga offers a wealth of benefits that can enrich every aspect of life. By embracing chair yoga as a holistic practice for well-being, individuals can embark on a journey of self-discovery, growth, and transformation that leads to a more vibrant and enriched life.

7.2 Chair Yoga in Community: Exploring Group Classes and the Social Benefits of Practicing Together

Chair yoga is not only a personal practice but also a communal experience that thrives in group settings. Group chair yoga classes offer a supportive environment where individuals can come together to practice, share experiences, and build connections, fostering a sense of community and belonging. Let's delve into the social benefits of practicing chair yoga together in a group setting:

1. **Sense of Belonging**:
   - Group chair yoga classes create a sense of belonging and inclusivity, providing participants with a supportive community where they feel accepted and valued.
   - Sharing a common practice with others can help individuals feel connected and understood, reducing feelings of isolation and loneliness.

2. **Supportive Environment**:
   - Group chair yoga classes offer a supportive environment where individuals can encourage and uplift one another on their wellness journey.
   - Participants often form bonds with fellow classmates, providing a source of encouragement, motivation, and accountability.

3. **Shared Experience**:
    - Practicing chair yoga in a group setting allows participants to share their experiences, challenges, and triumphs with others who understand and empathize.
    - Sharing a common practice creates a sense of camaraderie and solidarity, fostering a supportive community where individuals can learn and grow together.

4. **Social Connection**:
    - Group chair yoga classes provide opportunities for social interaction and connection, allowing participants to meet new people and build friendships.
    - Engaging in chair yoga together can lead to meaningful connections and lasting relationships, enriching participants' social lives and expanding their support network.

5. **Positive Energy and Atmosphere**:
    - The collective energy and enthusiasm of a group chair yoga class can create a positive and uplifting atmosphere that enhances the overall experience.
    - Practicing together in a group setting can inspire participants to push themselves further, explore new possibilities, and embrace their potential for growth and transformation.

6. **Sense of Community**:
    - Group chair yoga classes foster a sense of community that extends beyond the studio walls, creating a network of support and connection among participants.
    - Participants often develop a sense of camaraderie and solidarity with their fellow classmates, creating a supportive community where individuals can share, learn, and grow together.

7. **Celebration of Diversity**:
    - Group chair yoga classes celebrate diversity and inclusivity, welcoming individuals of all ages, backgrounds, and abilities to come together and practice.
    - Participants have the opportunity to learn from one another's unique perspectives and experiences, fostering a rich tapestry of diversity within the community.

In conclusion, group chair yoga classes offer more than just physical exercise; they provide a platform for social connection, support, and community building. By practicing together in a group setting, individuals can experience a sense of belonging, support, and camaraderie that enriches their overall well-being and enhances their quality of life. Whether you're a beginner or an experienced practitioner, participating in group chair yoga classes can be a rewarding and transformative experience that fosters personal growth, connection, and joy.

7.3 Beyond the Chair: Adapting Chair Yoga Principles for Use in Daily Life

Chair yoga principles extend far beyond the confines of a yoga studio, offering practical tools and techniques that can be seamlessly integrated into daily life, whether at work, while traveling, or in any other setting. By incorporating chair yoga principles into everyday activities, individuals can enhance their well-being, reduce stress, and cultivate a greater sense of balance and presence. Let's explore how chair yoga principles can be adapted for use in daily life:

1. **Mindful Breathing**:
    - Incorporate mindful breathing techniques into daily routines to promote relaxation and reduce stress. Take moments throughout the day to pause and focus on your breath, even if just for a few deep breaths.
    - Practice mindful breathing while commuting to work, waiting in line, or during moments of stress at work. Use the breath as an anchor to bring yourself back to the present moment and cultivate a sense of calm and clarity.

2. **Posture Awareness**:
    - Maintain awareness of your posture throughout the day, whether sitting at a desk, standing in line, or walking down the street. Sit and stand tall, with shoulders relaxed and spine aligned.
    - Use chair yoga principles to improve posture while working at a desk by adjusting the height of your chair, using a lumbar support

cushion, and taking regular breaks to stretch and move.

3. **Desk Yoga**:
   - Incorporate simple chair yoga stretches and movements into your workday to relieve tension and promote circulation. Stretch your arms overhead, twist gently from side to side, and roll your shoulders back and down.
   - Practice seated cat-cow stretches, neck rolls, and wrist stretches to release tension in areas commonly affected by prolonged sitting and typing.

4. **Mindful Movement Breaks**:
   - Take short mindful movement breaks throughout the day to refresh and re-energize. Stand up and stretch, walk around the office, or take a few moments to practice chair yoga poses such as seated forward folds or gentle twists.
   - Use mindful movement breaks as an opportunity to reset and refocus, allowing yourself to come back to your tasks with renewed energy and clarity.

5. **Stress Management**:
   - Use chair yoga principles to manage stress and promote relaxation during busy or challenging moments. Practice deep breathing, visualization, or progressive muscle relaxation to calm the nervous system and reduce tension.

- Take mini relaxation breaks during the day to step away from stressful situations and engage in calming activities such as deep breathing or mindfulness meditation.

6. **Travel Yoga**:
    - Adapt chair yoga principles for use while traveling to maintain a sense of well-being on the go. Practice deep breathing exercises, gentle stretches, and mindfulness techniques to stay grounded and centered during travel.
    - Use chair yoga poses and movements during long flights or car rides to alleviate stiffness and promote circulation. Stretch your arms, legs, and spine while seated, and take regular breaks to walk and stretch.

By incorporating chair yoga principles into daily life, individuals can cultivate greater mindfulness, reduce stress, and enhance overall well-being, regardless of their environment or circumstances. Whether at work, while traveling, or in any other setting, chair yoga offers practical tools and techniques for living a more balanced, mindful, and fulfilling life.

7.4 Lifelong Practice: Encouragement for Maintaining a Consistent Chair Yoga Practice for Lifelong Well-Being

Committing to a consistent chair yoga practice can have profound and lasting benefits for lifelong well-being. While it may be easy to start a new practice, maintaining it over the long term requires dedication, perseverance, and a sense of commitment to your own health and happiness. Here's some encouragement to help you stay on track with your chair yoga practice for a lifetime of well-being:

1. **Embrace the Journey**:
   - Understand that your chair yoga practice is a journey, not a destination. Embrace the process of learning and growing with each practice session, knowing that progress comes with time and consistency.
   - Celebrate your achievements, no matter how small they may seem. Whether you're improving your flexibility, finding more ease in a challenging pose, or experiencing greater peace of mind, every step forward is worth acknowledging and celebrating.

2. **Listen to Your Body**:
   - Honor your body's needs and limitations as you practice chair yoga. Pay attention to how you feel during and after each session, and adjust your practice accordingly to prevent injury and promote self-care.
   - Remember that your practice will evolve over time, and it's okay to modify poses or

take breaks as needed. Listen to your body's wisdom and trust yourself to make choices that support your well-being.

3. **Find Joy in the Practice**:
   - Cultivate a sense of joy and curiosity in your chair yoga practice. Approach each session with an open heart and a playful spirit, allowing yourself to explore new possibilities and experiences.
   - Focus on the present moment and savor the sensations of movement, breath, and awareness as you practice. Find moments of joy and gratitude in the simple act of being present with yourself and your practice.

4. **Set Realistic Goals**:
   - Set realistic and achievable goals for your chair yoga practice, taking into account your current level of fitness, mobility, and flexibility. Break larger goals into smaller, manageable steps to help you stay motivated and focused.
   - Celebrate your progress along the way, whether it's mastering a new pose, increasing your flexibility, or simply showing up to practice consistently. Recognize and appreciate the effort you're putting in to prioritize your well-being.

5. **Integrate Yoga into Daily Life**:
   - Look for opportunities to integrate chair yoga into your daily life beyond formal practice

sessions. Incorporate mindfulness techniques, breath awareness, and gentle movements into everyday activities such as sitting at your desk, standing in line, or walking around the house.

- View your chair yoga practice as more than just a physical exercise routine; see it as a way of life that permeates every aspect of your being, guiding you towards greater balance, harmony, and well-being.

6. **Stay Connected with Community**:

    - Stay connected with a supportive community of fellow practitioners who share your passion for chair yoga and well-being. Join group classes, workshops, or online communities where you can share experiences, learn from others, and draw inspiration and encouragement.

    - Surround yourself with positive influences and like-minded individuals who uplift and support you on your journey towards lifelong well-being.

Remember that consistency is key when it comes to reaping the benefits of chair yoga for lifelong well-being. By staying committed to your practice, listening to your body, finding joy in the journey, and staying connected with community, you can cultivate a lifelong practice that nourishes your body, mind, and spirit for years to come.

CHAPTER EIGHT

8.1 CELEBRATING YOUR JOURNEY: REFLECTING ON THE TRANSFORMATIVE POWER OF CHAIR YOGA FOR SENIORS

As seniors embark on their chair yoga journey, it's important to take moments to reflect on the transformative power of this practice and celebrate the profound impact it can have on their lives. Chair yoga offers much more than just physical exercise; it provides a pathway to greater well-being, vitality, and joy. Let's explore why it's essential to celebrate this journey:

1. **Physical Transformation**:
    - Chair yoga empowers seniors to reclaim their physical vitality and mobility, regardless of age or fitness level. Through gentle movements, stretches, and strengthening exercises, seniors can experience improved flexibility, balance, and strength, enabling them to engage more fully in their daily activities and hobbies.
    - Celebrate the milestones along the way, whether it's touching your toes for the first time in years, standing taller with improved posture, or feeling stronger and more resilient in your body. Each achievement is a testament to your dedication and perseverance.

2. **Emotional Resilience**:
    - Chair yoga cultivates emotional resilience and well-being by providing seniors with tools to manage stress, anxiety, and other emotional challenges. Mindfulness practices, breathwork, and relaxation techniques help seniors develop greater self-awareness, compassion, and inner peace.
    - Celebrate the moments of calm and clarity you experience during your chair yoga practice, as well as the sense of emotional balance and stability that accompanies regular practice. Recognize the strength and courage it takes to navigate life's ups and downs with grace and resilience.
3. **Mental Clarity and Focus**:
    - Chair yoga enhances mental clarity and focus, sharpening cognitive function and improving memory and concentration. Mindful movement, breath awareness, and meditation techniques help seniors cultivate a sharper mind and a greater sense of mental agility.
    - Celebrate the moments of clarity and insight you experience during your chair yoga practice, as well as the increased mental sharpness and alertness you feel in your daily life. Acknowledge the power of your mind to adapt, learn, and grow with each practice session.

4. **Spiritual Connection**:
   - Chair yoga offers seniors an opportunity to deepen their spiritual connection and cultivate a sense of purpose and meaning in life. Through practices such as meditation, visualization, and reflection, seniors can explore their inner selves and connect with something greater than themselves.
   - Celebrate the moments of awe and wonder you experience as you connect with your inner wisdom and intuition, as well as the sense of peace and fulfillment that comes from aligning with your deepest values and aspirations.

5. **Community and Connection**:
   - Chair yoga fosters a sense of community and connection among seniors, providing a supportive environment where individuals can come together to share experiences, learn from one another, and celebrate their progress.
   - Celebrate the bonds of friendship and camaraderie you form with fellow practitioners, as well as the sense of belonging and acceptance you feel within your chair yoga community. Cherish the moments of laughter, shared wisdom, and mutual support that enrich your journey.

By celebrating your chair yoga journey, you honor the progress you've made, the obstacles you've overcome, and the growth you've experienced along the way. Take time to acknowledge and appreciate the transformative power of chair yoga in your life, and let it inspire you to continue on your path towards greater health, happiness, and well-being.

8.2 Continuing the Path: Resources for Further Exploration

Embarking on a journey of chair yoga is just the beginning of a lifelong exploration of well-being and self-discovery. To deepen your practice and expand your understanding of chair yoga, consider exploring a variety of resources, including recommended reading materials and online resources. Here are some valuable resources to support your continued path:

1. **Books**:
    - "Chair yoga mastery series "by Henry I. Great. This series offers comprehensive guide offers a variety of chair yoga poses, sequences, modifications suitable for seniors over 55. Along with excellent and transforming tips for integerating chair yoga into everyday life.
    - "Chair Yoga: Sit, Stretch, and Strengthen Your Way to a Happier, Healthier You" by Kristin McGee: This comprehensive guide offers a variety of chair yoga poses, sequences, and modifications suitable for all levels, along with tips for integrating chair yoga into daily life.
    - "Chair Yoga for Seniors: A Gentle Sequence to Get You Started" by Lynn Lehmkuhl: This

accessible book provides a gentle chair yoga sequence specifically designed for seniors, with clear instructions and illustrations to support your practice.

- "Every Body Yoga: Let Go of Fear, Get on the Mat, Love Your Body" by Jessamyn Stanley: While not specifically focused on chair yoga, this empowering book offers insights into body positivity, self-acceptance, and finding joy in movement, which can be valuable for chair yoga practitioners of all ages and abilities.

2. **Online Resources**:
    - Yoga Journal (www.yogajournal.com): Yoga Journal offers a wealth of articles, videos, and tutorials on chair yoga, including pose breakdowns, sequences, and expert advice from experienced instructors.
    - DoYogaWithMe (www.doyogawithme.com): DoYogaWithMe features a selection of chair yoga classes suitable for all levels, from gentle stretches to more challenging sequences, led by knowledgeable instructors.
    - YouTube: Search for chair yoga videos on YouTube to find a variety of free resources, including guided practices, tutorials, and inspirational talks by leading yoga teachers.

3. **Online Courses**:
    - Udemy (www.udemy.com): Udemy offers a range of online courses on chair yoga for

seniors, beginners, and individuals with specific health concerns. Courses cover topics such as gentle stretching, relaxation techniques, and mindfulness practices.

- Yoga International (www.yogainternational.com): Yoga International provides online courses and workshops on a variety of yoga topics, including chair yoga, accessible yoga, and yoga for seniors. Courses are led by experienced instructors and accessible from anywhere with an internet connection.

4. **Local Classes and Workshops**:

    - Check with local yoga studios, community centers, or senior centers in your area to see if they offer chair yoga classes or workshops. Attending in-person classes can provide valuable opportunities for hands-on instruction, personalized feedback, and connection with fellow practitioners.

5. **Online Communities**:

    - Join online communities and forums dedicated to chair yoga or yoga for seniors to connect with like-minded individuals, share experiences, and ask questions. Websites such as Reddit (www.reddit.com) or specialized yoga forums can be excellent places to find support and inspiration on your journey.

By exploring these resources and continuing to engage with your chair yoga practice, you can deepen your understanding, cultivate new skills, and enrich your overall well-being. Remember to approach your practice with curiosity, openness, and compassion, and let your journey unfold with each breath and each moment on the mat.

8.3 Gratitude and Farewell: Closing Thoughts and Well Wishes for Your Ongoing Wellness Journey

As we come to the end of this journey through the transformative practice of chair yoga, I want to express my deepest gratitude for joining me on this path of self-discovery, growth, and well-being. Whether you're just beginning your chair yoga journey or have been practicing for years, I hope this book has provided you with valuable insights, inspiration, and tools to support your ongoing wellness journey.

As you continue on your path, I encourage you to carry with you the following sentiments:

1. **Gratitude for Your Body and Mind**:
   - Take a moment to express gratitude for your body and mind, recognizing their incredible resilience, strength, and capacity for healing. Approach your chair yoga practice with gratitude for the opportunity to nourish and nurture yourself from the inside out.

2. **Compassion for Yourself and Others**:
   - Cultivate a sense of compassion for yourself and others as you navigate the ups and downs of life. Embrace the imperfections and

challenges along the way with kindness and understanding, knowing that each experience offers an opportunity for growth and learning.

3. **Joy in the Present Moment**:
    - Find joy and fulfillment in the present moment, savoring each breath, each movement, and each sensation as you practice chair yoga. Let go of worries about the past or future, and fully immerse yourself in the richness of the here and now.
4. **Connection with Community**:
    - Stay connected with your chair yoga community, whether online or in person, drawing strength, inspiration, and support from your fellow practitioners. Share your experiences, insights, and challenges with others, knowing that you are not alone on this journey.
5. **Courage to Explore and Grow**:
    - Be courageous in your willingness to explore new possibilities, challenge yourself, and step outside your comfort zone. Trust in your inner wisdom and intuition to guide you as you continue to evolve and grow on your wellness journey.

As you move forward, may you continue to experience the profound benefits of chair yoga in body, mind, and spirit.

May you find strength, peace, and joy in your practice, and may it serve as a source of inspiration and empowerment in all areas of your life.

With deepest gratitude and warmest wishes for your ongoing wellness journey,

Conclusion

In conclusion, chair yoga offers a pathway to holistic well-being that is accessible, inclusive, and transformative for individuals of all ages and abilities. Throughout this book, we have explored the many facets of chair yoga, from its physical benefits of improving flexibility and strength to its profound effects on mental clarity, emotional resilience, and spiritual connection.

We've delved into the foundations of chair yoga, exploring its origins, principles, and techniques, and we've learned how to adapt chair yoga poses and practices to suit our individual needs and limitations. We've discovered the importance of mindfulness, breath awareness, and posture alignment in chair yoga, and we've explored how these principles can be integrated into daily life for greater vitality and well-being.

We've celebrated the power of chair yoga to enhance mobility, flexibility, strength, and balance, empowering individuals to live life to the fullest at any age. We've explored how chair yoga can be a source of relaxation, stress relief, and rejuvenation, helping individuals find peace and tranquility amidst life's challenges.

We've also recognized the social benefits of chair yoga, from fostering community and connection to promoting a sense of belonging and support among practitioners. We've explored how chair yoga can be adapted for use in various settings, from the workplace to travel, making it a practical and versatile tool for enhancing well-being wherever life takes us.

As we conclude our exploration of chair yoga, I invite you to carry the lessons and insights from this book into your daily life, embracing chair yoga as a lifelong practice for health, happiness, and fulfillment. May you continue to cultivate mindfulness, compassion, and joy in all that you do, and may chair yoga serve as a guiding light on your journey to holistic well-being.

Thank you for embarking on this journey with me. May your practice be filled with peace, love, and gratitude, now and always.

With warmest regards, *[Henry J. Great]*

THANKS FOR READING